Embracing
Special Needs Parenting
Your Child Needs a Good Parent

By: Maria Cruz & Patrick Baldwin

Copyright 2018
American Christian Defense Alliance, Inc.
Baltimore, Maryland
ACDAInc.Org

All Rights Reserved. No part of this publication may be reproduced in any form or by any means, including scanning, photocopying, or otherwise without prior written permission of the copyright holder.

Special Request

Thank you for purchasing our book and supporting our Ministry. We actually have two requests – To Pray for Our Ministry and to Read this Book All the Way through. No Ministry can Survive without Prayers and Support so we ask you to keep our Ministry in Your Daily Prayers and Pray as the Lord leads.

We encourage you to Read the Book you purchased all the way through. Many Books NEVER Get Read, and the ones that do only get read the first few pages.

One of our Special Request is that if you are serious about learning the material in this book that you take time to actually read this book in its entirety – all the way through.

We all lead such busy lives nowadays and can get side tracked so easily, please take a moment to consider my words and read to the end of the book and keep us in Your Prayers.

Thank You once again for purchase. We deeply appreciate Your Prayers and Support and know that God will Bless You as You continue to Bless this Ministry.

Table of Contents

Special Request.. 2

Embracing Pregnancy, Your Child, and Parenting.. 6

Chapter 1: Handle With Care 7

Chapter 2: The Miracle of Life 13

Chapter 3: Meant to be Parents...............18

Chapter 4: We're Having a Baby...............24

Chapter 5: The First Trimester 32

Chapter 6: The Second Trimester.............39

Chapter 7: The Third Trimester 46

Chapter 8: Let's Do This...........................53

Chapter 9: Family 58

Chapter 10: Children are the Future.........62

Parenting Special Needs Children............65

Prelude..66

Chapter 1: You Are Going to be the Parent of a Special Needs Child..........................67

Chapter 2: Guarding Your Heart, Soul, Mind, and Strength...74

Chapter 3: True Love is Devoid of All Pride 96

Chapter 4: Overcoming the Educational Obstacles..................................**105**

Chapter 5: We Are Family......................**111**

Chapter 6: Let Your "Light" Shine..........**116**

Chapter 7: Dealing With Special Social and Communication Needs **122**

Chapter 8: Dealing With Special Neurological Needs **127**

Chapter 9: Dealing with Genetic and Physical Special Needs..........................**133**

Chapter 10: Your Not-So-Secret Secret Thoughts **142**

Special Gift **146**

Stay in Contact......................................**148**

Find All Our Books.................................**149**

Additional Formats................................**151**

Embracing Pregnancy, Your Child, and Parenting

Your Guide Book to Learn How to Unlock the Secrets of Successful Parenting

By: Maria Cruz & Patrick Baldwin

Chapter 1: Handle With Care

Psalm 127:3 says, *Children are a heritage from the Lord, offspring a reward from Him.*

...from the LORD—that's where our children come from. The LORD. He entrusts them to us to care for; helping them go from infancy to adulthood safely, securely, and in an atmosphere that reflects God's love as much as is humanly possible.

There are a number of verses and passages of scripture in the Bible that reflect and teach this truth. We'll be looking at several of them throughout the pages of this book. I want to begin, however, by taking a look into the heart and mind of the woman I consider to be the most Godly mother of all times. Her name: Hannah.

We are introduced to Hannah in the first chapter of the Old Testament book of First Samuel. Hannah, who is one of Elkanah's two wives, is a tender-hearted and Godly woman who desperately longs to be a mother.

Her inability to conceive a child is something Peninnah, Elkanah's other wife, takes great pleasure in. Peninnah's taunting and ridicule plants seeds of insecurity and doubt in Hannah's mind; doubts that Elkanah quickly puts to rest; assuring his sweet wife that his love for her is true—child or no child.

I'm sure this had to bring at least some degree of comfort to Hannah's heart and mind, but it didn't change the fact that Hannah wanted to be a mom more than anything in the world. Hannah knew, though, that wanting to be a mom wasn't enough. Hannah knew that the gift of motherhood came from one 'place' and one 'place' only—God.

So Hannah prayed. She prayed and she prayed and she prayed some more. But her prayers weren't 'just' to become a mom. Hannah told God that if He would bless her with a child she would give the child back to him—literally. She told God that if He would bless her with a son she would give him to Eli to be raised up as the next High Priest and Judge over all of Israel.

After praying the prayer Hannah and Elkanah conceived a child. When the baby was born they named him Samuel. And true to her word, when Samuel was about three or four years old Hannah took him to live in the Tabernacle with Eli so that he could learn the duties of the priesthood. Samuel grew up to be a man of deep faith and one who obeyed God to the letter. He was the last Judge of Israel before they demanded that He appoint someone to be their king.

I'm sharing Hannah's story with you to remind you that your children are on loan to you from God. You are their caretakers and their role models. God has charged you with the task, aka, given you the privilege of overseeing some of His most priceless treasures.

As a steward of these treasures you need to be sure you care for them the way God expects you to—the way He told us to in Deuteronomy 6:5-9:

And thou shalt love the Lord thy God with all thine heart, and with all thy soul, and with all thy might. And these words, which I command thee this day, shall be in thine heart: And thou shalt teach them diligently unto thy children, and shalt talk of them when thou sittest in thine house, and when thou walkest by the way, and when thou liest down, and when thou risest up. And thou shalt bind them for a sign upon thine hand, and they shall be as frontlets between thine eyes. And thou shalt write them upon the posts of thy house, and on thy gates.

You are to teach them diligently. When you teach diligently you teach consistently; meaning on a regular basis. But teaching with diligence also implies that you are meticulous and careful to make sure they don't just know *about* God, but that they know who God *is*—His character.

God doesn't just tell us the manner in which we are supposed to teach our children. No, God also gives us the specifics of how to get the job done.

He tells us to **talk of them when thou sittest in thine house, and when thou walkest by the way.** He goes on to say we are to teach our children when they lay down and when they are awake. In other words, the Word of God is to permeate our children's lives. Their exposure to God's Word needs to be the norm—not the exception. We are to **teach our children to see God** in everything, **give thanks** to God for all things, **give God the credit** He is due, and **give God total control** of our lives.

And then He gets to the really personal part. Teaching our children these things needs to be done by example. Children really do learn what they live, and God is calling us to make sure they live in homes where God is first and foremost every day and in every way.

That's a pretty tall order—an awesome responsibility. It is not impossible, though, because God never gives you a job to do without also providing you with the resources necessary to do it…and do it well.

The Word of God ...prayer...the Holy Spirit...Godly counsel from other parents...a parent-heart that wants to give their children the best life possible—these are the resources we have at our disposal.

You need to know, however, that these resources aren't meant to be optional. Deuteronomy 6 isn't a suggestion or a wish. It is a command from the creator to the moms and dads He entrusts with His most priceless treasures.

Hannah knew she was raising Samuel *for* God. Raising your children *for* God is your job, too.

Chapter 2: The Miracle of Life

Have you ever looked at a newborn baby? I mean really looked—their tiny fingernails, the perfect little curvatures of their ears, the soft little eyelashes, the way they instinctively know when Mom is nearby? They are pure perfection, aren't they? They are also a living, breathing miracle.

Yes, life is a miracle. It couldn't just happen by accident. Too many things have to be just right in order for an egg and sperm to get together and stay that way. Oh, I know there are those first-time-I-had-sex-I-got-pregnant people out there. But they are far from the norm. In fact, the UK's Daily Mail website and the New York Post newspaper reported that research conducted on three thousand couples showed that on average, it takes couples one hundred and four sessions of lovemaking before pregnancy is achieved.

Additional research shows that less than half of all couples get pregnant within the first six months of trying to conceive, but that just over ninety percent conceive within a year. So like I said, there's nothing accidental or coincidental about it.

I also know that getting the news that you are expecting can take you on a rollercoaster of emotions. Excitement, disbelief, anxiousness, fear, awe, surprise, elation…and sometimes disappointment and anger are the most common.

Not every pregnancy is planned or desired. Most teenagers aren't trying to achieve pregnancy when they're in the back seat of a car or home alone on the couch. Sometimes couples don't feel ready to start a family for one reason or another, but find out they are anyway. Other couples feel their families are complete and/or are getting ready to be empty-nesters when suddenly….

For others—especially couples who have experienced the grief of miscarriage or infertility—pregnancies can be scary. They want it so badly they are too afraid to let themselves enjoy it. They don't want to get their hopes up only to have their hearts broken again.

And then there are those that count down the days from the time their chances of conceiving were the highest until they can take a pregnancy test to see if this will be the month.

No matter what you are feeling or thinking, though, you need to know that God knows exactly what's going on and he knows exactly what He is doing. He knew wayyyyyyyyy back when he said, "Let there be light…" when each of us would be conceived. I know that's a lot to wrap your head around, but it's true. The Bible says so in Psalm 139:15-16:

My frame was not hidden from You, When I was made in secret, And skillfully wrought in the lowest parts of the earth. Your eyes saw my substance, being yet unformed. And in Your book they all were written, The days fashioned for me, When as yet there were none of them. (NKJV)

Every mother out there can testify that giving birth and being a parent is truly a gift from God – The Miracle of Life if you would. Hopefully God will see fit in His plan to bless you abundantly with children in the near future. Just remember Children have angels assigned to watch over them so make sure you're gracious to strangers.

Hebrews 13:2 says, "Do not forget to show hospitality to strangers, for by so doing some people have shown hospitality to angels without knowing it."

As far as I know I've never welcomed an actual angel into my home, but I have been the recipient of their God-given ability to intervene in my life in a way that still leaves me 'on my knees thankful'.

Remember: Babies aren't made by accident. A mommy and daddy's perfect timing doesn't even guarantee anything. It is God's perfect timing that results in the miracle of life.

Chapter 3: Meant to be Parents

Genesis 1:27-28 says, *"So God created man in His own image; in the image of God He created him; male and female He created them. Then God blessed them, and God said to them, "Be fruitful and multiply; fill the earth and subdue it; have dominion over the fish of the sea, over the birds of the air, and over every living thing that moves on the earth."thing that moveth upon the earth."*

Genesis 9:1 says, *"So God blessed Noah and his sons, and said to them: "Be fruitful and multiply, and fill the earth."*

In Genesis 28:3, Isaac said to Jacob, *"May God Almighty bless you, And make you fruitful and multiply you, That you may be an assembly of peoples;*

And finally, Psalm 127:3-5 tells us, *"Lo, children are an heritage of the Lord: and the fruit of the womb is his reward. As arrows are in the hand of a mighty man; so are children of the youth. Happy is the man that hath his quiver full of them: they shall not be ashamed, but they shall speak with the enemies in the gate."*

It isn't difficult to see the common thread running through these four verses, is it?

God wants us to be parents. Next to worshipping Him and sharing the message of the Gospel to anyone and everyone we possibly can, being a parent is the most important job God gives us to do. Remember: the job of parent is synonymous with being the caretaker of God's most precious and priceless treasures...children.

Unfortunately, not every parent knows just how important their job is. If they did, the National Children's Alliance wouldn't have to report that over 700,000 children in the US are treated or receive some type of service because of abuse or neglect each and every year. Additionally, over 3 million children in this country are the subject of an intervention or protection order.

Why do you think this is? Why would anyone want to harm an innocent child? The answers to that question are varied. Some would say it is because the parents were abused or neglected, so they don't know any better. Others would say it is because these parents is not mature enough to be a parents. And still others would say that an abusive parent's actions are beyond their control because of an addiction or emotional/mental disorder. While these things may or may not be true, the real reason child abuse/neglect happen is because God is not present in the home. When God is absent from a home a lot of other things are absent, as well.

Things like patience, gentleness, genuine selflessness, diligent teaching about God, and unconditional love.

As Christians we need to be conscientious about making sure God is present in our homes. We have the same perspective on parenting that God designed us to have. We need to make sure we embrace our role as parents; viewing it as a praiseworthy responsibility rather than a chore. It is a praiseworthy responsibility we need to take to heart.

Some would ask then, if being a parent is something God desires us to do, then why are there Christian couples suffering from infertility? And if being fruitful and multiplying is so important, then where does that leave couples who don't want children or those who don't marry? Are they living outside of God's will for mankind?

Infertility is an emotionally and physically painful condition. But know this...infertility is NOT a sin and it is NOT God's way of punishing someone. Infertility is a medical condition caused by a number of different things. What's more, infertility doesn't mean you cannot be a parent. Adoption is always as possibility. The process isn't always easy and (take it from someone who knows) it is considerably more labor-intensive than having a biological child. And don't let anyone ever tell you that adoptive parents aren't parents in every sense of the word, because they are.

Choosing to be childless is not a sin, either. Christian couples choose to remain childless in order to be able to pursue their ministries without the distractions of family. Frank and Ella are an example of this mindset.

Frank and Ella spent thirty years as dedicated youth directors. Neither felt comfortable or working with small children or babies.

Tweens and teens, however, were a different story. They poured themselves into ministering to young people this age and their efforts were highly effective. So rather than having biological children of their own, this couple chose to 'have' dozens of children over the years; loving, teaching, and mentoring them to know and love the LORD. Other couples may choose not to have children for any number of reasons that are personal in nature; reasons that are between them and the LORD. For anyone to pass judgement on these people would be very wrong.

According to scripture God prefers we have children. Children are proof of the love between a man and a woman. Children are the hope of the future—both the future of this world and of the Church. So be fruitful and multiply; raising your children to know the LORD and that they are fearfully and wonderfully made by Him and for Him.

Chapter 4: We're Having a Baby

You've been anxiously waiting for the days and weeks to pass so that you could take a pregnancy test. The day came, you took the test, and you are on 'cloud nine' because the test came back positive. YOU ARE GOING TO HAVE A BABY!

In the days immediately following, you and your spouse shared the good news with family and close friends. You've pinched yourself (literally or figuratively speaking) a few times to remind yourself you aren't dreaming—that this is actually happening. You and your spouse have already started tossing a few names around and you have already had your first mini-panic-attack over whether or not you can go through the labor process and then actually be responsible for a helpless baby. If so, relax. All of these thoughts (and a whole lot more we're getting ready to talk about) are completely normal.

They are just part of the whole pregnancy experience. Your thoughts and worries are no different than those of any other parent-to-be, so we're going to spend the next few minutes talking about the most common thoughts and concerns of parents during those first few days and weeks following the moment you find out that you are going to have a baby.

Telling your spouse

It wasn't all that long ago women didn't have the capability to find out whether or not they were pregnant until they were at least eight weeks into the pregnancy or without going to the doctor to have blood drawn to test to see if the level of the hormone, hCG is high; indicating there is a pregnancy.

It also wasn't all that long ago expectant fathers weren't nearly as involved in the pregnancy experience or the birth of their baby as most expectant fathers are today.

Expectant fathers were usually unaware pregnancy was even a possibility until their wife shares the good news.

Today things are a lot quicker, easier, and a lot more of a joint effort. The prospective parents communicate a lot more directly about the possibility of whether or not pregnancy is possible. If, however, you are an expectant mom who wants to surprise your husband with the wonderful news, there are a number of fun ways to do so.

Give your husband a baby onesie with the logo of his favorite sports team, and a note that says 'from' your baby saying can't wait to meet you Dad, a giant cookie with your approximate due-date written in icing, or a devotional book for dads - nice.

Telling your family and close friends

Your parents, grandparents, and siblings should hear the news before the general public does. A phone call or face-to-face visit to share your good news may be a bit 'plain', but it gets the job done. If you want to spice it up a bit try gifting grandparents with a t-shirt or mug with a grandparent saying on it is always fun. Phone calls, emails, or posts on your social media are effective and sufficient for telling friends and extended family members about your pregnancy.

Telling your employer

A close friend of mine had to go to her new boss the second day she was on the job and tell him she was pregnant. The pregnancy was something she and her husband had all but given up on happening, so learning she was going to be a mother again was an answered prayer.

But it was also nerve racking. She didn't know her new employer so she had no idea how he would take the news. Thankfully he was gracious and understanding and did not treat her any differently than he did any other employee.

Telling your employer should be a priority. They need to know so that you can discuss how things like prenatal appointments and maternity leave are handled. You also need to talk to the HR person to find out what your insurance does and does not cover—what your options are regarding participating providers.

While there are some jobs that might require you to go to a limited duty status or make some special arrangements for bouts of morning sickness, being on your feet too long, or other such things. You need to remember that being pregnant is not a disease or a disability. Don't treat it as such by taking advantage of your coworkers or employer.

Choosing an OBGYN

More than likely you already have a doctor who will care for you throughout your pregnancy and who will deliver your baby. You have probably been seeing them for your yearly exams. But there are instances in which this is not the case. If for example you have to move for a job just prior to giving birth – you will need to find a new doctor.

The whole doctor situation can be a bit unnerving. You want someone you can trust, right? Someone you feel comfortable with. Because this isn't always possible it is just one more reason for you to put your faith in the Great Physician—Jesus. He is always on-call. He will never be too busy to care for you. He knows your every need and those of your baby. He is the one you can always put your trust in and know He's got your back.

Early good prenatal care is essential

No matter who your doctor is or how and when you tell everyone else about the baby growing inside of you, the most important thing you can do for yourself and your baby is to take great care of yourself physically and emotionally.

Thankfully, most expectant moms don't have any trouble tweaking their normal lifestyle or routines once they find out they are expecting. You know—things like giving up caffeine, bouncing over rough and rocky trails on an ATV, or even putting their hobby of refinishing antique furniture on hold.

I'm here to suggest, however, that you start these things before you know you are pregnant. If you are trying to get pregnant you want to create the most welcoming, healthy, and conducive environment for your growing baby as possible.

So if you are reading this book in anticipation of the day you find out you are pregnant, start making those changes today. If you are newly-pregnant there is no question that the things I mentioned above (along with several others) are no-no's for pregnant women wanting a healthy pregnancy and healthy baby. But if there are somethings you are in question about, don't hesitate to ask your doctor.

Congratulations! This is a wonderful, special, and amazing time in your life. Enjoy it. Make it among the happiest months of your life.

Chapter 5: The First Trimester

This book combines the biological and physiological aspects of pregnancy with the spiritual aspects of pregnancy. So in addition to learning or being reminded of what is taking place inside you (or your wife) I am also going to provide you with Scriptures of encouragement and reminders that your baby is a treasure in God's storehouse of treasures, and in spite of all that He created, He sees each and every single one of us as priceless... irreplaceable...one-of-a-kind.

Fertilization

"Do you know the time when the wild mountain goats bear young? Or can you mark when the deer gives birth? Can you number the months that they fulfill? Or do you know the time when they bear young? ~Job 39:1-2

In spite of the fact that you may be planning to try to become pregnant by charting your ovulation times, the fact remains that there is only One who knows the moment fertilization takes place and a new life begins. That One is God.

Within those first few hours when the egg and sperm join together, a new life is formed that contains chromosomes from each parent. These chromosomes determine the sex of the baby along with a host of other things – but those things I'm sure you may already know about so let's move on . . .

The earliest stages of formation

For You formed my inward parts; You covered me in my mother's womb.
~Psalm 139:13

Looking at a picture of a three week-old baby may not provide a very clear picture of what is going on inside, but wonderful things are happening.

By the end of the third week after conception, your baby's body is basically three layers of cells that are working hard to form various intricate parts of the body. The first layer of cells forms the skin, the body's nervous system, and their eyes and ears. The second layer is what grows to become the baby's heart (along with the rest of the circulatory system), their bones, muscles, and ligaments, their kidneys, and their reproductive system. The inner-most layer of cells forms the respiratory and digestive organs and systems.

A brain, spine, arms, and legs

I will praise You, for I am fearfully and wonderfully made, Marvelous are Your works, And that my soul knows very well. ~Psalm 139:14

Four weeks after your baby has been conceived, which is usually around the time most women find out they are pregnant, they are starting to develop a brain, the spinal column is forming, and arms and legs look like little buds ready to sprout to be fully infant-sized.

Your baby is growing and developing their most important parts for living a healthy, well-rounded life. This is just another reason you need to make sure you are taking proper care of yourself so that your baby receives the best of care, too.

Accepting the Child God Gives You

For the body is not one member, but many. If the foot shall say, because I am not the hand, I am not of the body; is it therefore not of the body? And if the ear shall say, Because I am not the eye, I am not of the body; is it therefore not of the body? If the whole body were an eye, where were the hearing?

If the whole were hearing, where were the smelling? But now hath God set the members every one of them in the body, as it hath pleased him. ~1 Corinthians 12:14-18

Weeks five and six following conception are busy ones, to say the least. The shape of the head becomes more distinctive, as do the eyes, ears, and nose. While your baby cannot yet see, the retinas are forming; meaning and it won't be long before they can.

Fingers begin to form on the little short arms that are still yet to grow to their full length. The upper lip is formed, and the neck becomes straighter and more distinguishable.

Most amazingly of all (in my opinion, anyway) is the fact that all of this is happening to a little person about the size of a penny!

During the final weeks of the first trimester your baby's size goes from that of a penny to about the size of a credit card. By the time the first trimester comes to an end your baby also has toes, elbows, definite eyelids, buds inside the mouth that will eventually become baby teeth, red blood cells are being produced by the liver (yes, that's there, too), and their genitalia begins to make its presence known on the outside of the body.

No wonder you don't feel like your normal self

Now if God so clothes the grass of the field, which today is, and tomorrow is thrown into the oven, will He not much more clothe you, O you of little faith? "Therefore do not worry, saying, 'What shall we eat?' or 'What shall we drink?' or 'What shall we wear?' For after all these things the Gentiles seek. For your heavenly Father knows that you need all these things..
~Matthew 6:30-32

Now that you've been given a very brief and basic rundown of what is going on inside a woman's body during those first weeks of pregnancy, do you even have to ask why they don't feel like themselves? Is it any wonder that extreme fatigue is completely normal for expectant mothers, as is nausea, aka morning sickness?

These first weeks and months can be physically and emotionally exhausting. There's no doubt about that. But as a Christian you have the promise that God can and will sustain you through this time so that you can enjoy the blessings of being a steward of one of His treasures.

Chapter 6: The Second Trimester

As you enter into the second trimester of your pregnancy, you usually begin to feel better (no more morning sickness) and your energy level begins to rise. For many women, the second trimester of pregnancy is a time when they feel better than they've ever felt. They are excited about the baby's upcoming arrival. They are enjoying the fact that they are growing a baby-bump; bringing with it all sorts of positive attention and well-wishes. Thinking about names, nursery décor, and all the other fun things that go with becoming parents seem to start taking root during the second trimester.

While everything going on, on the outside is great, what's happening on the inside is even more thrilling. Let's take a look...

Diapers not needed...yet

As you do not know what is the way of the wind, Or how the bones grow in the womb of her who is with child, So you do not know the works of God who makes everything.. ~Ecclesiastes 11:5

Beginning around the eleventh week after conception (which is technically the thirteenth week of pregnancy because the two weeks between ovulation and what would have been your next period are counted) your baby begins to pee. Their pee becomes part of the amniotic fluid your baby will live in until they makes their grand appearance into the world.

Along with that major developmental milestone, your baby's bones are hardening, more red blood cells are forming in other organs, and their sex organs are becoming more distinctive.

Something new almost every day

Before I formed thee in the belly I knew thee; and before thou camest forth out of the womb I sanctified thee, and I ordained thee a prophet unto the nations. ~Jeremiah 1:5

As you progress further into your second trimester your baby starts developing more and more of the functions and characteristics they will need to live outside the womb. They develop the ability to hear, blink their eyes, and their heart is pumping around one hundred pints of blood each day. Your baby is also rolling and flipping around quite a bit, but is still too small for you to feel these movements. Don't worry, it won't be long before you do. Additionally, their digestive system is now working and they are almost as long as a dollar bill.

Reaching the halfway mark

But the very hairs of your head are all numbered. ~Matthew 10:30

During the second trimester you will hit the half-way mark of your pregnancy. It is about this time that an ultrasound can reveal to you the sex of your child (if you want to know).

Being able to recognize your baby as either a boy or a girl isn't the only significant milestone in your baby's development during this time though. Throughout the remaining weeks of the second trimester of your pregnancy you will begin to feel your baby's movements. This is one of the most exciting aspects of pregnancy. To be able to feel your baby moving around inside your body is…is…well, there really are no adequate words to fully capture the specialness of how this feels (physically or emotionally).

It is also possible for the baby's father, grandparents, or whoever else you invite, to feel the baby's movements by placing your hand on your tummy during the baby's more active times. This, too, is a very special event and a precious bonding experience for husbands and wives and for soon-to-be-dads and their unborn child.

Discovering the sex of your baby and being able to feel their movements isn't the only things that happen during these final weeks of the second trimester. There are also many significant things going on inside your baby's body.

The sound of your voice

My son, hear the instruction of thy father, and forsake not the law of thy mother: For they shall be an ornament of grace unto thy head, and chains about thy neck .~Proverbs 1:8-9

Your baby has definite times of being asleep and awake. They can even be awakened by your movements and noises outside the womb. I find this incredible, don't you!

Your baby's body is covered in the cheesy coating and a fine layer of fuzz or hair. These things both serve to keep your baby's skin from being chapped by the amniotic fluid.

Your baby's fingerprints and footprints are engraved onto their little bodies. Each one, we know, different from anyone else's every born.

Your baby can suck their thumb and recognize Mom's voice. Yes, that's right—*they know your voice before they ever see your face!*

By the end of the second trimester your baby's lungs are developing at a rapid pace; preparing them to make their grand entrance in a few months.

But because the baby's lungs and their ability to suck properly are not yet fully established, it is important that you take care to keep your baby from making their entrance too soon to avoid complications. If that happens, however, just remember God is the One in Control and He has a plan for everyone including your baby.

By the time you come to the end of your second trimester your baby weighs approximately two pounds and is approximately nine inches long – and that to me is just Awesome to think about.

Chapter 7: The Third Trimester

You're almost there—'there' being the end of your pregnancy. At this point you are feeling both excited and nervous. You are getting tired of wearing maternity clothes, yet are 'certain' you'll never be able to wear anything a 'normal' woman wears again. You have days you feel energized and ready to take on the world, but then others you feel like a beached whale that can barely get one foot in front of the other. It's that whole rollercoaster effect kicking into high gear again.

This is also the point in your pregnancy when you begin getting serious about preparing the nursery, enjoy putting all those tiny little clothes in the closet and dresser drawers, and preparing for maternity leave from your job.

At this point you also need to be finalizing arrangements for childcare once you return to work—if you plan to do so. I cannot stress how important this is, because the weeks you are home with your baby after he or she arrives fly by all too quickly. In other words, you aren't going to have the time or desire to deal with this issue while on maternity leave, so it is essential you do so now.

I also want to tell you how important it is to *enjoy* these last few weeks of your pregnancy. These are special weeks in your life—weeks that cannot be replicated no matter how many children you have. Each pregnancy story is different and needs to be experienced as the miracle it truly is.

Getting ready, but not quite set to go

For we are his workmanship, created in Christ Jesus unto good works, which God hath before ordained that we should walk in them.
~Ephesians 2:10

The third and final trimester of your pregnancy is your baby's time to develop and grow into all those finishing touches that make us capable of living outside the womb. During these last few weeks your baby's hair comes in on their heads or not(it just depends on your family).

Your baby is also stretching and kicking—sometimes causing you a good deal of discomfort. For example, one mom delivered her second daughter with an extremely bruised tailbone—bruised from the inside due to the baby's near-constant kicking and jabbing –ouch! And then there are those more comical incidents surrounding the baby's movement during the last trimester. More than one expectant mom I know has had a bowl of popcorn or other snack resting on her belly, only to have it knocked off by the baby's movements.

Your baby can and will likely have hiccups; something you can feel them doing, but cannot help them with.

At the onset of the third trimester your baby will also start working quite diligently to put on weight. The added weight and layers of fat they form fill out their skin making it less wrinkled and protects their hardening bones. This protection is necessary, because even though their bones are hardening, they are still quite soft in comparison to what they will be later on. Remember—they have to be pliable enough to make it through the birth canal.

The Father's finishing touches

The spirit of God hath made me, and the breath of the Almighty hath given me life. ~Job 33:4

Thirty weeks after conception (week thirty-two of your 'official' pregnancy) your baby starts breathing practice. They are gearing up for the outside world. To this point they have breathed in and out, but it has been more instinctive than purposeful.

At this point in time the bulk of the fuzz that has covered your baby's body also begins to fall off. The degree to which this happens varies greatly in each child. As you may already know, some babies are more hairy than others when they are born. Premature babies are especially so, if born before this stage of development. The amount of baby fuzz isn't an indicator of anything being wrong with the baby. It is simply just one aspect of their unique nature showing through.

In the final weeks of gestation your baby develops the ability to detect light. They gain about an ounce of weight per day, the added weight and fat content causes their little bodies to fill out even more, and they begin positioning themselves into the birth canal.

Your doctor will likely be checking you weekly at this point to make sure everything is going as it should.

Some doctors even do an ultrasound toward the end of the pregnancy to check to make sure the umbilical cord isn't wrapped around the baby's neck, to make sure the baby's head is not so large that they feel it would be unsafe for the mother to have a vaginal delivery, and a number of other things.

It is also at this point that mothers who are having a c-section will schedule their baby's delivery. Most c-sections are scheduled to take place the week of the due date or possibly a few days prior to the due date the mother was given. This is done in an effort to avoid the baby trying to come on its own, which in most cases of mothers having C-sections, would not be a good thing.

Most C-sections are done for the sake of either the mother or child's physical condition. However, if at all possible I strongly recommend having a vaginal birth as there are many added health benefits for the baby.

Remember, the last stages of your baby's development are important to you and to them. So continue to take care of yourself and to give your baby every possible opportunity to grow and develop the way God intended them too.

Your third trimester (and pregnancy) is almost over. D-day is fast approaching.

Chapter 8: Let's Do This

At this point in your pregnancy you probably have the crib set up, you've been to childbirth classes (if you chose to take them), you have your bag packed for the hospital, and a solid birthing plan in place. You know exactly how you want things to go and you have every intention of making the birth of your child an absolutely, positively, perfectly wonderful experience.

The only thing you aren't counting on is the fact that more often than not, the best laid birthing plans fly right out the window about the time the contractions start coming around five minutes apart.

This really hurts

To the woman He said: "I will greatly multiply your sorrow and your conception; In pain you shall bring forth children; Your desire shall be for your husband, And he shall rule over you."
~Genesis 3:16

With the first baby you 'know' it's going to hurt. You've talked to other moms. You've read a few books and watched a few movies. But geez, how hard can it really be? If it was *that* bad there wouldn't be as many babies as there are. If it was *that* bad, not even sex would make it worth the 'risk'.

The thing to remember is that every women is different and every birth is different. When my wife started getting contractions I thought it was false labor and went back to sleep because I had exams the following day. However, shortly thereafter she came back in, woke me up, and said "Its Time to Go". We contacted the OBGYN and got everything we needed and headed out.

When she got to the hospital she was close to 5cm dilated. My wife no doubt is a solider and not every women could handle that as if it was no big deal but there are some.

Keep in mind my wife is just over 5' tall and weighs a little over 100lbs (not including the pregnancy weight). So if she can do it you probably can too. Just don't have any preconceived ideas about how much pain it will be because you truly don't know.

The experience of giving birth is not something you can plan for right down to your baby's first cry. There are too many variables you have no control over. Things like: where you are when your labor starts, how long the labor and delivery will take, how cooperative your baby is, how well you work with your body's natural instincts to get the job done, and the overall type of labor experience you have.

If you are reading this and think that because you are about to give birth to baby number two, don't get too smug. Every birth is different. Don't believe me? Ask any mom who has more than one child.

That thing they say about the pain being worth it...they're right

A woman, when she is in labor, has sorrow because her hour has come; but as soon as she has given birth to the child, she no longer remembers the anguish, for joy that a human being has been born into the world. ~John 16:21

I'm not going to spend a lot of time talking about the actual labor and delivery process or about the things that take place within the first few hours and days following your child's birth. Your doctor will cover all of that, and that's as it should be.

What I do want to say is that becoming a parent truly is a cause for joy and celebration. It really is the most amazing and most important thing you will ever do in this world—second only to giving your life to Christ.

So will you really forget the pain? Will the memory really go away?

The Word of God is true in all ways—including this. Though you will remember that it hurts and your memories of the event will always be there, the memories will be such that you will see the marvelous good that came from it—not the anguish and suffering you felt.

Chapter 9: Family

Welcoming a new baby into your family is news parents don't hesitate to share while having a big smile plastered across their face and heart. Think about it...how many birth announcements have you gotten that say something like, "We're as happy as we can be to announce we are now a family of three!" or "Our family is growing day by day now that baby number three has come to stay."?

Parents, grandparents, aunts, uncles, cousins should all be a part of your child's life for so many reasons. There are far too many to cover them all adequately, lets take a few minutes to cover the most important ones now...

Family provides a sense of belonging

God set up the institution of family because He knows we thrive best when we have the communion of relationships. He knows we need to be needed and need to be wanted. He knows family units and provides the sense of belonging He created us to want and need.

Family brings a sense of responsibility

Having a child changes you—or at least it should. Having a child causes you to be less selfish and more selfless. You suddenly find yourself completely and utterly responsible for another human life. You realize that what you do and how you do it affects someone else. You realize that where you go, how you act, what you say, and everything else about your life isn't just about you—it's about you and your baby.

Family becomes more important

How many new parents have you heard say something to the effect that when their baby was born their own parents (the baby's grandparents) suddenly became wiser and smarter than they'd ever been before?

News flash! The grandparents didn't suddenly become anything (other than grandparents). The wisdom and knowledge was there before the baby was born. But when faced with the awesome and daunting task of actually being a parent themselves, well….

The role of grandparent, aunt or uncle can be a precious resource in the lives of children and their parents. For a child, these extended family members can be sounding boards, people who have time when parents don't, an added source of encouragement and unconditional love, someone to teach them skills their parents don't have, someone to just hang out with, someone to whom they can give back all of these things, and someone they can look up to as an example of faith.

Those of you who have families that can bring these things into your child's life should be thankful for the blessing of family. It is something you should not take for granted and should not deprive your child of.

Those of you who do not have family to lean on and glean from, do not have to miss out completely. You can 'adopt' a family in your church. There are undoubtedly people as hungry for a family as you are. Family isn't always about blood and DNA. It's about exhibiting the kind of love that says "I love you just because". Never forget those that claim the name of Jesus Christ and claim His Blood are Adopted into the Family of God – So You are NEVER Alone!.

Chapter 10: Children are the Future

Babies and children just add that something extra into a family's dynamics. They bring a sense of innocence, wonder, fun, and youthfulness into a home. Children also give us purpose—or at least they should. Being a parent should make you stand a little taller on the 'ladder' of integrity. They should make you think on your words before you speak them; making sure they are honest, kind, and fair. Children should make you walk a straighter path; working hard, spending your money wisely, being honest and forthright, and setting a solid example of how to live. Children should make you desire to know God more fully and to teach them to know God on a personal level, too, because children are the future of society and of the Church.

One of the most heart-rending statements I've ever heard went something like this: The worst possible feeling a parent could have is the feeling that they might not spend eternity with their children in heaven.

Ouch! That cuts deep, doesn't it? As parents we need to be mindful of the fact that we are responsible for raising our children to know the LORD and to have a desire to seek his purpose for their lives.

That being said, you need to remember that your purpose is to raise them to know these things—not live their lives for them.

We have this Promise from God . . . .

Train up a child in the way he should go, And when he is old he will not depart from it.
~Proverbs 22:6

While none of us are perfect; meaning we all make parenting mistakes (and plenty of them), if we do our job to raise our children as directed by God in the Bible, we have nothing to worry about. You can do it as God fearing Parents that seek the Living God and honor Him by following the Word of God on how to raise your children.

Don't let things discourage or frighten you, along the way. There will always be ups and downs in life but in all things God is an ever present help in a time of need – Trust in Him, Allow His Word to inspire you to become a great parent who raises awesome kids.

Do as we are told in Lamentations 2:19...

Arise, cry out in the night: in the beginning of the watches pour out thine heart like water before the face of the Lord: lift up thy hands toward him for the life of thy young children that faint for hunger in the top of every street.

In reading this book you have either learned or have been reminded of the fact that being a parent isn't just something physical that you do. Being a parent is also a spiritual act—one that God intends to be a spiritual act of worship aimed at Him.

God knows that when we see our children as the priceless treasures they are we will love, nurture, and cherish them in such a way that glorifies God.

Parenting Special Needs Children

A Christian Guide to Parenting Children with ADHD, Autism, Asperger's, and other Psychological, Behavioral, or Physiological Disorders

By: Patrick Baldwin

Prelude

Having worked for close to 20 years with those in our society that are considered some of the most vulnerable, I wanted to write this book to offer Biblical Guidance for the Christian Parent.

Often times we may become overwhelmed with the thoughts, responsibilities, and day to day grind that having a special needs child can bring to your life. It is critical to see Your Child through the Eyes of God and to Keep Your Focus on Jesus Christ along the Way.

I truly Pray that this book will be a Blessing to You and Your Family and hope that You will share it with other Christian Parents who may be also dealing with the challenges of Parenting a Special Needs Child.

God Bless You

Chapter 1: You Are Going to be the Parent of a Special Needs Child

When we see the little line on the pregnancy test saying there is a baby growing inside of you, the last thing you probably think about (or one of the last things) is whether or not your baby will have special needs when it comes to their physical, mental, or emotional wellbeing.

You aren't thinking about whether or not you will be able to afford special equipment they might need to live. You aren't thinking about what your insurance will and won't cover and what kind of help you can get to make up the difference. You aren't thinking about whether or not your house will 'work' for a wheelchair, if your boss will allow you to work from home or how you will juggle work and five or six doctor's appointments a month (or possibly in a week).

You aren't thinking about the fact that your baby—the one you've just 'met'—is one of the millions of children in this country that will receive some form of special education when he or she goes to school. And that's providing he or she can go to school.

No, you aren't thinking about those things at all. You are thinking about whether the baby is a boy or girl, when the due date will be, who to share the happy news with first (other than your spouse, of course), and you even start rolling possible names around in your mind. In other words, your thoughts are focused on the joy that comes from bringing a new baby into this world.

Well guess what? Bringing a new baby into this world regardless of whether or not they have special needs *is* a joy. Each and every tiny little life that takes their first breath after working their way into this world is a cause for celebration and joy *because* we are all fearfully and wonderfully made by the LORD God, our Creator.

Nevertheless, learning your child has special needs—whether you find out prior to or immediately after their birth, or a few months or years down the road—is difficult. Your love for your child instinctively wants them to be 'normal'. You don't want them to have to struggle. You don't want them to have to go through the experience of feeling different from the rest of the kids or to experience the loneliness often felt from being left out of so many things kids like to do. You don't want to see the hurt in their eyes and know their hearts are breaking when they are made fun of or ostracized by their peers.

What's more, you can't help worrying about how their condition or circumstances is going to affect your life and the lives of other family members. And then you start feeling guilty for feeling and thinking that way; making you even more anxious.

Am I right? You know I am. But the GREAT news is that it is perfectly normal and okay to feel and think these things—as long as you are near enough to Jesus to dump it all at His feet so that he can replace all of those things with what you need in order to do the very special job you have been given by God to do.

That's right—being given the responsibility of parenting a child with special needs is NOT a form of discipline or punishment. Instead, God is saying, "I have a special job for you because your heart's capacity to love and nurture is above and beyond what is normal. I created you with the ability to see beyond the obvious into the heart and soul of one of my children, so I need you to raise them up for me."

We see this truth in the Gospel of John, chapter nine, when Jesus heals a man who had been born blind. Jesus and His disciples were coming into a village when they saw the man, who was most likely begging in front of the marketplace or along the road that led into the village.

When the disciples saw that he was blind, they asked Jesus whether it was he or his parents whose sin had caused him to be born blind. (That's the punishment 'thing' I just mentioned.)

Jesus immediately replied that neither the sins of the man nor those of his parents had caused his blindness. And then in the next breath, Jesus added these words: Jesus answered, "Neither this man nor his parents sinned, but that the works of God should be revealed in him..." (John 9:3 NKJV)

Did you get that? The man's blindness wasn't a curse or punishment. He had been born blind so that he could be an instrument through which Jesus' holiness and power could be displayed. He was literally a partner in Jesus' ministry!

So while parenting a special-needs child maybe wasn't what you anticipated doing as a parent, and while you may feel completely overwhelmed and even terrified at the prospect of doing so, don't let these feelings rob your child of the joy he or she deserves to feel in your touch and see in your eyes that says, "I'm so glad you are mine." And whatever you do, don't let these feelings rob you of the joy you deserve to experience in becoming and being a parent and of the blessing of being God's partner in showing the world just how Holy and Mighty He is.

Bible Verses to Encourage You

And not only that, but we also glory in tribulations, knowing that tribulation produces perseverance; 4 and perseverance, character; and character, hope.
~Romans 5:3-4

And the Lord said unto him, who hath made man's mouth? or who maketh the dumb, or deaf, or the seeing, or the blind? have not I the Lord? ~Exodus 4:11

For thou hast possessed my reins: thou hast covered me in my mother's womb. I will praise thee; for I am fearfully and wonderfully made: marvelous are thy works; and that my soul knoweth right well. ~Psalm 139:13-14

Lo, children are an heritage of the Lord: and the fruit of the womb is his reward. ~Psalm 127:3

Chapter 2: Guarding Your Heart, Soul, Mind, and Strength

You can have all the joy, joy, joy, joy down in your heart, in your head, and bubbling up out of your soul imaginable but that won't erase the fact that parenting a special-needs child is hard work. It is physically exhausting, mentally and emotionally draining, time-consuming, and often times very, very lonely. I think it's safe to say that this is one of those things about which your grandma would say, "The most worthwhile jobs we do are the hardest jobs we do".

Because there is so much required of you, it is important that you take care of yourself. *Good* care of yourself. This is something many parents of special-needs children don't do a very well. Generally speaking, parents put the needs of their children in front of their own needs—as we should in many instances, but not *all*.

And when you take into consideration that the demands on your life because of the increased needs of your child.... I guess you could say that parents of special-needs children have some special needs of their own.

What you are about to read is a list of things you need to be doing for YOURSELF. Don't make excuses and the words "I can't" are not allowed—not even in your head or under your breath. Taking good care of yourself is key to doing your job to the best of your ability and key to knowing you, too, are fearfully and wonderfully made (Psalm 139).

1: Spend time in the Word daily

Ten or fifteen minutes spent reading the Bible each day is food for the soul, body, and mind. Don't just focus on the Psalms or the Gospels—books of the Bible that are usually viewed as the 'feel good' books of the Bible. While you *do* need to make them part of your Bible study, they shouldn't be the only part.

When you spend time in the books of history you become more grounded and sure of the fact that God does have a plan.

The books of Job and Ecclesiastes humble you and remind you that the most important things in life aren't things and that God really does have the whole world (including you and your child) in His hands.

The book of Esther gives us an extra dose of courage and reminds us that our ultimate purpose is to bring Glory to God through all we do and say.

The prophets don't spare words. They tell it like it is when it comes to reminding us that we are all sinners. But they are equally eloquent when it comes to reminding us of God's abundant love and mercy—love and mercy we can draw on every...single...day.

James and most of Paul's letters are the books that keep us on the straight and narrow. They define Christian character, warn us of the consequences for living outside of God's laws and expectations, and reaffirm the promises of heaven in all its glory when we abide in Jesus Christ.

Read God's Word. Apply it to your life. Let it speak to you. Let it change you.

2: Pray

One of the biggest concerns and complaints of parents with special-needs children is that they don't have many people they can talk to who really 'gets' it. Not on a regular basis, that is, because the parents who *do* 'get' it are as busy as they are. But God always hears and He is always available. No, He's not someone you can sit around the table with over a cup of coffee or someone you can chat with while you take a lap or two around the block. But He *is* there, He *does* listen, and He *does* care.

You also need to know (or be reminded of the fact) that your conversations are not one-sided. God responds to you. He responds by:

- Telling the Holy Spirit what to say to you (Jon 16:13)
- Speaking to you through the Scriptures
- Providing answers through your conversations and interactions with others – Something called Confirmation.

In 1 Thessalonians 5:17 we are told to pray without ceasing. If you do that, you'll also be conversing with God nonstop.

3: Eat a healthy diet

God created our bodies to operate at optimum efficiency and capacity when we feed our bodies a steady diet of the food He created for us to eat. Meat, fruits, veggies, dairy products, grains...the things He created to fuel our bodies.

Sure there are exceptions—food allergies and personal tastes, for example. But for the most part you really need to make sure your diet consists primarily of foods free of chemicals, dyes, and processing.

If you are still looking for things like chips, blooming onions, mocha latte caramel coffee with an extra shot of caffeine, diet soda, and seven-layer lasagna on the list of best foods, you can stop. They aren't there. They never will be.

Eating a healthy diet keeps your body working the way it should. Your heart is healthier. Your body doesn't produce a lot of bad fat for you to carry around. You think more clearly. You reduce your risk of getting things like heart disease, diabetes, kidney failure, and bone and joint disorders due to carrying around too much weight. You have more energy. Your immune system does a better job of fighting off colds and the flu.

Question: What's not to like about the benefits of eating a healthy diet?

Answer: Nothing. So do it!

4: Get plenty of exercise

If your child has physical limitations that require you to bathe them, dress them, and help them move from one place to another, you are undoubtedly getting quite a bit of physical activity. But that doesn't mean you don't need to get twenty minutes or so of walking, yoga, aerobics, or whatever else you like to do at least three days a week.

If at all possible, you should also set aside an hour or two each week for more rigorous exercise. A few possible options include: Water aerobics, tennis, volleyball, working out at the gym, swimming laps, or anything else you enjoy that gets your heart pumping.

The physical benefits of exercise go without saying and should be reason enough to make sure you get this time each week. But the physical benefits are just the tip of the proverbial iceberg. So what are the benefits?

- Exercise increases oxygen to the brain; helping you clear your head and think more rationally and clearly.
- Exercise releases endorphins. Endorphins are hormones that send messages to the brain that tell the brain to think positive thoughts. Endorphins also lessen our perception of pain. They intercept the signals from our nerves and send the message to the brain that it doesn't hurt as bad as 'all that'.
- Exercise keeps your weight in check and your heart healthy.

- Exercise gives you some much-deserved time off from your responsibilities as a parent. Even if it is only for a few minutes a day, it is worth it.
- Exercise boosts your immune system. This is actually one of the top two or three reasons parents of special-needs children take time to exercise. After all, when parents get sick (especially Mom) chaos at home can quickly ensue. So remember… "An ounce of prevention is worth a pound of cure".
- Some forms of exercise provide you with a social outlet. Even if you and a friend take several laps around the block or park, it still counts as time you can enjoy conversations without interruptions.

5: Date nights and marriage protection

Couples with children—no matter how many and no matter what their needs are—all run the risk of letting parenting, work, money-matters, and everything else push their marriage and its wellbeing to the backburner. But when you add the stresses of raising a special-needs child to the mix, the chances of this happening increase significantly.

The financial burdens that come from having a special-needs child are often very heavy to bear. The primary caregiver (usually Mom) doesn't have a lot of time to just sit and talk. She doesn't always have the luxury of prioritizing how her time is spent. That is usually done for her out of sheer necessity. That's why as parents of a special-needs child you need to make conscious and consistent effort to have couple time free of ANY talk about home, money, the kids, or anything else that pertains to your daily routine.

You need to make a conscious effort to make romantic gestures and let your spouse know they are second only to God.

What? But...our child needs me to do…. Who has time for romance? And since my life pretty much revolves around making sure our kids are taken care of, there's not really much else to talk about.

Oh, but there is. There is plenty to talk about:
- Make plans for a weekend getaway...just the two of you
- Talk about an upcoming event at church
- Talk about some things you would like to make time to do for yourself
- Make plans for a family weekend
- Talk about current events
- Recall memories from your dating years and the early years of your marriage

- Talk about the reasons you love one another
- Talk about long-range goals for your marriage and family
- Talk about something funny you saw on television or at the grocery store
- Make a list of ideas of things you can do to keep your marriage fresh and thriving...and then start doing the things on that list

There are several other things you need to make sure you don't neglect to do in order to keep your marriage safe and fresh. These things include:

- Worshipping together.
- Serving together in your church and community.
- Letting your children see and hear you being (appropriately) affectionate with each other.
- Not allowing your children to play you against one another.

- Making sure you kiss each other good morning, hello, goodbye, and goodnight.
- Telling each other "I love you" every single day.
- Not neglecting your appearance—your 'Sunday best' isn't always necessary, but baggy pants, t-shirts, and a messy-hair-don't-care look doesn't say much about the way you feel about yourself. And if you don't care about yourself, it's hard for other people to do so.
- Taking care of your body.
- Showing an interest in your spouse's job (in and away from the home).
- Making their friends feel welcome in your home.
- Respecting their need for 'me' time and giving them that luxury.

- Making sure 'me' time and 'friend' time never add up to more than the time you spend with your spouse and your family.
- Living with the attitude of submission (for wives) and sacrificial love and leadership (for husbands) as directed in the New Testament book of Ephesians.

7: Fellowship

You need fellowship. You need to spend time with your peers; studying God's Word, socializing, enjoying recreational activities and outings, and just hanging out. Just being yourself.

While there is nothing wrong with part of this fellowship coming in the form of support groups or play groups with other parents of special-needs children, this should not be your *only* outlet.

These groups are can be very beneficial—a lifeline for many of you—but you need to be able to fellowship in ways that address *your* needs and interests...not your child's.

Don't think this is being selfish. It's not. By giving yourself this time you are giving your family a better and you—an energized, more confident, refreshed you. So don't feel guilty about taking some time for a Bible study, a weekly game of golf or tennis, meeting up for coffee and fellowship, a book club, or some other group where you can share your passion for your hobby with others who feel the same.

The amount of time you allow yourself isn't a number that is set in stone. There is no magic number that guarantees your needs will be met. For some, an afternoon, evening, or possibly an entire day (or most of it, anyway) a week is doable. For others, though, an hour or two a week is a priceless and treasured gift that happens only with a great deal of planning, preparation, and help from others.

Speaking of help...

8: Ask for help

You can't do this on your own. Physically...emotionally...mentally...you need help and support.

The help and support you receive can come from a number of different resources. Some of these resources exist solely for the purpose of helping parents of special-needs children and the children themselves. Other sources of help are people who love and care about you and want to be the hands and feet of Jesus in your life. And you need to let them do that.

Bobby and Shannon were the parents of six year-old twins and a three year-old born without hands—his arms stop just below his elbows. Bobby, Shannon, and all three children are completely comfortable with their life.

Even the twins are a great help when it comes to feeding, dressing, and playing with their little brother. But they are hesitant to leave their son in anyone's care other than his grandparents when they came to visit or the physical therapist they met with a couple of hours a week. So other than these two hours a week and four or five visits a year from grandparents, Bobby and Shannon took no time for just the two of them.

Friends from church have offered to take all three of the kids on numerous occasions, but Shannon always made an excuse. Thanks, but no thanks, was the message she conveyed. But then one day, a middle-aged woman at church asked Shannon a question that stopped her in her tracks. She asked, " Why do you insist on keeping people from doing what Jesus wants them to do?"

"Excuse me," Shannon asked back, somewhat offended. "What do you mean?"

"People in this church, including me, want to be part of your family and want you to be part of ours. We want to minister to your family, get to know you and your kids, let you know you have people who love and care about you. We want to live and love the way Jesus told us to, but you won't let us," was the woman's answer.

Shannon didn't know what to say. She'd never thought about it like that before. She was so focused on not wanting to appear to be a charity case or give people a reason to think they needed to feel sorry for them and their son, that she had completely forgotten that Jesus calls us to love and serve one another. This woman was right! By not accepting their offers for help and fellowship, they were robbing these people of opportunities to be like Jesus. And what's more, they were robbing themselves of the blessings that come with being a part of a family of believers.

From that day on Shannon and Bobby were more than happy to take people up on their offers to babysit so they could have date nights. And they were equally happy to return the favor by doing the same for other young families in the church. Josephine (the woman who talked to Shannon) and her husband became surrogate grandparents to their children, and relationships were built that will undoubtedly last a lifetime.

Today Shannon and Bobby are the parents for four and grandparents to two. They are also in charge of a parent's night out ministry at their church, because they know what it is like to need help AND they know how important it is for others to be able to offer it.

Besides your church family, other possible resources for help include:

- Healthcare agencies
- Playgroups for children with physical disabilities
- Daycare facilities that cater to children with special needs
- Friends and neighbors
- Support groups (for emotional and mental help you need)

9: Me time

In addition to the time you spend with just your spouse and time spent with your friends and peers, you need to have a few minutes of 'me' time every day. Thirty minutes or so each day to do whatever you want to do by yourself. Take a walk. Soak in the bathtub. Read a book. Bake cookies. Shoot some hoops. Watch television without interruption. Surf the web. Catch up on social media. Do your nails. Take a nap. Whatever you enjoy doing…do it.

The purpose of this time of solitude is to allow you to clear your head and not think about anyone or anything but yourself and what you are doing. This is your time to dream, plan, rest, relax, and even be a bit selfish.

Taking this time each day is so important. Knowing you have this time to look forward to each day helps you keep things in the proper perspective. It prevents you from feeling like you've lost your identity as an individual.

You are God's child. You are a spouse. You are a parent. You are an instrument of God's plan. Your body is the temple of the Holy Spirit. You cannot be and do these things if you are not practicing good self-care, so do it. It is your duty to yourself, your family, and to your God.

Bible Verses to Encourage You

It is vain for you to rise up early, to sit up late, to eat the bread of sorrows: for so he giveth his beloved sleep. ~Psalm 127:2

*I will both lie down in peace, and sleep;
For You alone, O Lord, make me dwell in safety.
~Psalm 4:8*

For I have satiated the weary soul, and I have replenished every sorrowful soul. ~Jeremiah 31:25

There remaineth therefore a rest to the people of God. For he that is entered into his rest, he also hath ceased from his own works, as God did from His. ~Hebrews 4:9-10

Chapter 3: True Love is Devoid of All Pride

Every parent's desire is to make their child's life good, happy, pleasant, and as carefree as possible. And why not? Isn't that just part of what loving someone is all about? But when you have a child with special needs, your quest to give these things to your child usually comes with a few (or a lot) more challenges.

Every parent is charged by God with the task of keeping their children safe and healthy, providing them with food, clothing, and shelter, and loving them unconditionally; nurturing and cherishing them for the treasure they are. Additionally, parents are responsible for raising their children to:

- Learn to be confident and comfortable with who they are
- Know that we are to be God-pleasers...not people-pleasers
- Recognize sin for what it is and rise above it

- To strive to achieve their goals and dreams

But again, children with special needs have to work a little harder to get the job done, and as their parent, *you* have to work a little harder to help them. Your success in doing so depends on your ability to set aside any prideful feelings you have—consciously or subconsciously.

Denial is not uncommon when you first learn that your child has special needs. These feelings are not necessarily evidence of shame or embarrassment. More often than not they stem from guilt, concern, and apprehension.

- Did I do something...or not do something that caused this?
- Will my child be able to enjoy at least some of the things a child should?
- Can I be the parent my child needs and deserves?

The reason for the feelings isn't necessarily important. What *is* important is that you set them aside for the sake of everyone involved. Don't let pride keep you from dong what is best for your child.

Early intervention

Denial has been the reason for many children's conditions and disabilities to go undiagnosed as soon as they could and should be. If your child isn't diagnosed as having special needs, then the problem isn't really there, right? Wrong! Early intervention often makes the difference in how severely their disability affects their life (and yours) and the degree to which they can function.

Parents, pretending or burying your head in the sand accomplishes nothing good. So don't deny your child every chance possible to be high-functioning and/or to receive therapy that allows them to be more mobile and independent. Get help at the first sign that a problem exists.

Your pediatrician will be able to connect you with available resources and information for your particular situation. Make use of them.

Living realistically

Once you know what your child's condition is and what their needs are and will be you need to listen intently and carefully to those who can point you in the right direction to get you and your child the help available to you. When meeting with therapists, doctors, and anyone else involved in your child's care, you might not always like what you hear.

Sometimes parents feel the plan of action isn't aggressive enough. Some feel it is too aggressive. And some think the medical community is too pessimistic in their outlook. These are the parents that believe if their child tries hard enough they can overcome their disability.

EXAMPLE: Jared's mom was thoroughly convinced that putting her son in a classroom for special-needs students that he would never reach his full potential. She believed that if he was in a traditional classroom setting he would work harder to be on a level 'playing field' with the rest of the class.

The problem with this line of thinking is that by putting expectations on Jared he simply cannot meet makes him feel bad about himself and causes him to doubt his ability to succeed. It's like giving a five year-old keys to the car and expecting them to be able to drive.

Your child has enough to deal with because of their special needs. Don't add to that by trying to make them someone they are not and by insinuating that you are ashamed of them or that who they are is not reason enough to love them with your whole heart. Accept the fact that they have limitations. Accept what those limitations are. Put them in a position to excel to the best of their ability. Celebrate their accomplishments. Love them for who they are.

Be your child's advocate and biggest fan

Today's children are only the second or third generation of children to not be hidden away or ignored just because they have special needs. Prior to this, children with special needs were considered to be disposable and less valuable than their 'normal' peers. Children with special needs and disabilities were often placed in institutions where they did little more than exist. Others were kept at home, but were not allowed to go to school and had little or no social interaction. Think: Boo Radley in *To Kill a Mockingbird*.

Thankfully, though, not every parent 'back then' thought or felt that way...

Neal and Bonita knew something was wrong with their second-born son, Gary, before he turned six months old. He wasn't meeting the developmental milestones for babies his age. But in those days and in their small town, it wasn't easy to get a correct diagnosis. When they did, the words they heard were MULTIPLE SCLEROSIS.

Neal and Bonita were encouraged to put Gary in a 'home' where he could live out his days (which they were told would be less than twenty years) peacefully and out of the harsh and unaccepting public eye. But they didn't want to put their son away. They knew God didn't make a mistake when he made Gary. They knew he was as treasured and loved as anyone else God created. They also knew that every child with special needs was one of God's precious treasures, too.

So with nothing but a determination and passion for wanting to help Gary and others like him to reach their full potential, Neal and Bonita recruited teachers and people who practiced a trade to work in what would now be called a sheltered workshop.

Gary is now an eighty year-old man who has never walked on his own, never ran, played catch, or spoken a word that is understandable by an 'untrained' ear. But he *has* appeared before three different presidents of the United States to champion for the rights of people with disabilities, gone to Europe to compete in the Special Olympics, won multiple gold and silver medals in the same, accumulated dozens of bowling trophies, and encouraged countless people just by being himself. But these things were possible only because his parents were his biggest fans and they championed for him with relentless energy, passion, and love.

Don't let anyone make your child feel worthless and unlovable. Believe in them and do whatever you can to make sure they are given every possible and feasible opportunity to reach their full potential.

Bible Verses to Encourage You

For I know the thoughts that I think toward you, saith the Lord, thoughts of peace, and not of evil, to give you a future and a hope. ~Jeremiah 29:11

Now unto Him that is able to do exceeding abundantly above all that we ask or think, according to the power that worketh in us... ~Ephesians 3:20

For we are His workmanship, created in Christ Jesus unto good works, which God hath before ordained that we should walk in them. ~Ephesians 2:10

Chapter 4: Overcoming the Educational Obstacles

Back in the day there was an ad campaign targeting high schoolers in an effort to convince them to pursue a college education. The campaign's slogan was, "A mind is a terrible thing to waste". And it's true, a mind *is* a terrible thing to waste—and that means your child, too.

Depending on where you live, your child's school may or may not be equipped to offer your child the educational resources they need and deserve. This is not something you should waste time being angry or bitter about. In most cases the lack of resources is due to a lack of money and/or a lack of qualified teachers in the district—neither of which will be changed by your anger or bitterness. Instead, be pro-active and take matters into your own hands. Instead of wasting your time and energy, put it to use by either becoming the resources your child needs or by going beyond the walls of the school to get them.

Here are some possible ways you might do that:

Depending on your child's special needs you might consider homeschooling your child. Or better yet, consider forming a homeschool coop with other special need's parents. This has proven to be especially helpful to both parents and students with needs such as dyslexia, mild autism, sensory problems, auditory processing disorder, and a variety of delayed development issues. Educating your child in this type of environment allows them to:

- Learn in a less congested environment with fewer distractions and risks of over-stimulation and more personalized attention
- Feel safer and more accepted among their peers
- Receive instruction and training at a pace and in a format that will allow them to thrive and excel

As for parents, working together shares the workload, provides a community of support and encouragement, and it allows you to know you are giving your child the learning environment most conducive to their learning style and capabilities.

Hire a tutor. Homeschooling on any level is not always possible. And quite frankly, it is not always the best route to take. Depending on your child's needs and the resources they have available in their school, you may find that by hiring a tutor your child will be able to stay on course with the mainstream student population. You don't need to go through a professional service to find a good tutor, though. Retired teachers, teachers who have opted to stay home with their own children, but who are willing to tutor a few hours a week, or college students in need of extra money are all great resources. A tutor gives your child the one-on-one they so often need to get them over the hump and to give them the moral support and encouragement to keep trying.

Specialized schools are available in some areas—usually large cities. These are somewhat expensive, however, but *do* offer the best in special-needs education. If you live near one of these schools don't let the price tag scare you. Funding is sometimes available through scholarship programs or organizations to aid and assist children with special needs.

Public schooling is free and available to children with mild to moderately-severe special needs. Many public schools have excellent programs for children with learning disabilities and a staff of loving, caring, and dedicated teachers. Often time's public schools also offer and allow personal aides or assistants for special-needs students. The job of a personal aide/assistant is to be their student's constant companion throughout the day; assisting them in whatever ways they need assistance.

Some of the things they might do include:

- Reading to them if they cannot read but can comprehend
- Signing for the deaf
- Writing for those that cannot write but are fully able to comprehend and can speak the answers
- Feeding and other personal care

No matter what educational obstacles you encounter or what path you choose for your child, remember...a mind is a terrible thing to waste.

Bible Verses to Encourage You

How much better is it to get wisdom than gold! and to get understanding rather to be chosen than silver! ~Proverbs 16:16

Take firm hold of instruction, do not let go; Keep her, for she is your life.
~Proverbs 4:13

Give instruction to a wise man, and he will be yet wiser: teach a just man, and he will increase in learning. ~Proverbs 9:9

Chapter 5: We Are Family

When asked what challenges a special-needs child brings to the dynamics of a family, the answers are all over the map.

- "I don't think of my child's needs as something that challenges our family," one parent said. "Being a family means seeing one another as equally valuable and loving one another for who we are. So if who we are, is someone who needs help eating or who cannot play ball, then so be it."
- "I find myself working harder than I really need to sometimes to make things equal for my kids. Sometimes I feel guilty about spending more time with my daughter because of her needs, but then God reminds me that not having to do those things for my boys is a good thing."

- "It is challenging. My now-seven year-old was three when an accident left her with some physical disabilities and mild learning disabilities. I was expecting our second child at the time, so adjusting to all the changes in our routine and life in general really did keep me from enjoying my new baby. I am constantly second-guessing myself in regards to how good a mom I am to each of them."
- "I leave for work every morning knowing my wife is on a non-stop schedule. I feel guilty for being gone so much, but our son's medical expenses are over the top. We'll never be able to see the light at the end of the tunnel. We would like to have another child, but don't know how in the world we could handle two.

- We want to know what it's like to parent a child that doesn't need round the clock care (or close to it). We want to know what it's like to go to our kid's ball game or dance recital. Is that so bad or wrong?"

- We have two boys in school and our four year-old son is low-functioning autistic. The six and nine year old boys are great with him at home, but I've noticed lately they get embarrassed when Judson acts out in public and they say things like, "Can't you just take us and Mom and Judson stay home?" Or "Judson can't do that, so why does he have to come?" I know some of that is natural, but right now I'm really struggling with how to teach my boys to love their brother for who he is and to love him like they love each other."

I could say all sorts of things on how I feel or what I think on how to handle the possible challenges a special-needs child can bring to your family. But what I think and how I feel aren't important. What is important is what God has to say on the subject of family unity...regardless of the physical, mental, or emotional issues that might be present. So take a few minutes to let God's Word soak into your heart and mind. Share these verses with your spouse, your children, and even your extended family members in an effort to remind them that we are ALL created in the image of God and are ALL equally loved and valued by him.

Bible Verses to Encourage You

Love suffers long and is kind; love does not envy; love does not parade itself, is not puffed up; does not behave rudely, does not seek its own, is not provoked, thinks no evil; does not rejoice in iniquity, but rejoices in the truth; bears all things, believes all things, hopes all things, endures all things ~1 Corinthians 13:4-7 (NKJV)

We love him, because he first loved us.
~1 John 4:19

Better is a dry morsel with quietness,
Than a house full of feasting with strife.
~Proverbs 17:1

For as we have many members in one body, but all the members do not have the same function, so we, being many, are one body in Christ, and individually members of one another. ~Romans 12:4-5

For the body is not one member, but many. If the foot shall say, because I am not the hand, I am not of the body; is it therefore not of the body? And if the ear shall say, because I am not the eye, I am not of the body; is it therefore not of the body? If the whole body were an eye, where were the hearing? If the whole were hearing, where were the smelling? But now hath God set the members every one of them in the body, as it hath pleased him. ~1 Corinthians 12:15-18

Chapter 6: Let Your "Light" Shine

Remember reading about Neal and Bonita and how they refused to stifle their son, Gary's potential in time when that was the norm for kids like Gary? Thankfully things are much different today.

Today parks have playgrounds for children with even the most severe disabilities.

Today public buildings have rams and entryways that are accessible to people in a wheelchair.

Today public restrooms are equipped with facilities with enough room to maneuver around in and with sinks, toilets, etc. placed at the right height.

Today even campground shower houses have wheelchair-accessible showers.

Today parking lots provide spaces for vehicles with special-needs drivers or passengers.

Today special-needs children can grow up to be special-needs adults who contribute to society in a positive manner by working, volunteering, and just living life to the fullest.

All of these things are definitely improvements over what used to be, but that doesn't mean life for families of special-needs children is not without its share of obstacles in their communities and their social lives.

When it comes to meeting and overcoming the challenges of special-needs children and their families in the community and on the social 'scene', you need to respond the same way you should when it comes to your child's education. You need to be a pro-active advocate instead of an angry, bitter parent. And the best way to do this is to help the world see what an amazing and precious person your child is.

Proverbs 31:8 (NKJV) says: *Open your mouth for the speechless, In the cause of all who are appointed to die.* So do it! Open your mouth, use your hands to open doors, your feet to walk through them, and your mind to think of ways to help your child be a part of the world around them. Don't hide their light under a basket. Let them shine for all those around them to see...and be blessed.

- Attend church and let your child be involved in the youth program to the extent they are capable of. Be willing to act as a chaperone for youth events so that your child can participate.
- Volunteer with your child. Taking their specific needs into consideration, consider participating in walk-a-thons (or wheel-a-thons, if necessary). Fill shoe boxes with gifts for other children. Ring the Salvation Army bells. Hand out personal care bags to the homeless. Visit a nursing home together.
- Join a play group.

- Visit the park on a regular basis.
- Enroll your child in swimming lessons, bowling lessons, or some other type of activity they are capable of participating in. *Many of these activities/lessons offer special lessons for children with various handicaps.
- Join 4-H, scouts, or another similar type of organization.
- Go to the weekly story hour at your library.
- Participate in free movie nights, craft-making events, kid-friendly lectures and demonstrations, etc. offered in your community.
- Go for ice cream or an occasional dinner at a favorite family pizza place or restaurant.
- Get them involved with Special Olympics.

The "Bible Verses to Encourage You" segments in previous chapters have already listed Exodus 4:11 and Psalm 139:13-14, but I want us to look at them again because they are important reminders to everyone that God creates each of us in his image and with a distinct set of purposes in mind. Special-needs children are not mistakes. God doesn't make mistakes. Special-needs children are special-*purposes* children and as their parents you need to help them accomplish those purposes in this world.

Bible Verses to Encourage You

And the Lord said unto him, who hath made man's mouth? or who maketh the dumb, or deaf, or the seeing, or the blind? have not I the Lord? ~Exodus 4:11

For thou hast possessed my reins: thou hast covered me in my mother's womb. I will praise thee; for I am fearfully and wonderfully made: marvelous are thy works; and that my soul knoweth right well. ~Psalm 139:13-14

But indeed, O man, who are you to reply against God? Will the thing formed say to Him who formed it, "Why have you made me like this?"
~Romans 9:20

Chapter 7: Dealing with Special Social and Communication Needs

Children with social and communication special needs are those with autism, Asperger, and ADHD (as well as a few others). But then you already know that, don't you? You know that your child has difficulties interacting socially and communicating their thoughts and needs.

The severity of these conditions varies widely from person to person. In some children it is a matter of controlling their intake of certain foods and providing them with a structured environment so that they don't feel (and act) like a loose cannon. But for others, the problem is much more intense. Some children cannot speak or communicate on any level. Some children cannot handle even slight changes in their routine without becoming unsettled and sometimes nearly impossible to manage or console. But again, you already know these things.

What you don't know...or need to be reminded of is that neither you nor your child is alone in the struggles you are facing to deal with life as you know it. God is ever-present.

His presence is visible in the words of the Bible:

He healeth the broken in heart, and bindeth up their wounds. ~Psalm 147:3

It is of the Lord's mercies that we are not consumed, because His compassions fail not. They are new every morning: great is thy faithfulness. The Lord is my portion, saith my soul; therefore will I hope in Him. The Lord is good unto them that wait for Him, to the soul that seeketh him. ~Lamentations 3:22-25

But God commendeth His love toward us, in that, while we were yet sinners, Christ died for us. ~Romans 5:8

Another means by which God proves His presence is in providing resources and counsel for you and your child. Because God has worked through others, we know that parents of children with autism and ADHD can help their child when they:

- Provide a consistent routine and schedule for their child
- Make home a safe, fun, and hazard-free place to be
- Make time for fun; doing things THEY enjoy doing
- Reward positive behavior
- Discover their child's triggers for tantrums and melt-downs and then take necessary actions and precautions
- Know the child's sensitivities (smell, sound, etc.) and try to avoid them or forewarn them
- Concentrate on the child's strengths; allowing them to achieve and excel

- Teach older children to use public transportation, tech gadgets, and other helps in order to be more independent
- Teach them to respect themselves
- Teach them to love, honor, and obey the LORD

Parents of children with Asperger's can help their children by:

- Help your child practice appropriate reactions to common social situations at home so they can learn without feeling judged or on display.
- Teach your children the meaning of common phrases that aren't meant to be taken literally, since many children with Asperger's are quite literal. Example: Telling a child with Asperger's that he is silly will often get this type of response: "I'm not silly, I'm Max."

- Give your child a safety phrase—something to say that will alert you that they are feeling anxious and scared and unsure of how to respond or react.
- Prevent situations when possible rather than try to cure them after the fact.
- Plan ahead and keep your child informed of what they can expect. Surprises and the unexpected are NOT enjoyable to them.
- Don't argue with your child. Negotiate or end the conversation until both of you are better able to communicate rationally.
- Let them 'run with' the things that interest them and don't try to squelch their methods of imaginary play.

Whatever level of function your child has, remember this: They are precious in God's sight and are significant to His plan.

Chapter 8: Dealing With Special Neurological Needs

In an effort to encourage you to stay the course and keep things in their proper perspective, I want to offer you a list of tips and suggestions for dealing with the special needs of your child in a way that will benefit them and the rest of your family. Remember: Every child deserves to know, beyond a doubt, that the only reason you *need* to love them is because they are yours—that's enough to merit your unconditional love.

Keeping that in mind, here are some things you can do to help your child with sensory processing disorder:

- Slow down. A lot of times children will be able to accept and enjoy new experiences if they are allowed to approach them at a slower pace.
- Give them space. Again, they need time to adjust to their surroundings and assess them in their own way.

- Keep things as visual as possible, as kids with sensory disorders are usually calmed by what they can see.
- Keep a bag full of items to distract your kids from sensory overload handy at ALL times.
- Be sensitive to their thoughts, feelings, and needs. Don't force things on them that aren't necessary.
- Introduce new sights, sounds, textures, and smells in a positive manner. Teach them to try something new, but let their response be the indicator of how far to take it.
- A therapy or specialized play group can be beneficial. Sometimes positive peer pressure works for the good of your child.

Children with auditory processing disorder:

- Should receive instructions in short, simple sentences. One step at a time.
- Should always be spoken to when facing them and when you are sure you have their attention.
- Keep things as visual as possible. Use chore charts, to-do lists, etc.
- Ask questions like: "Do you understand?" "Do you know what you are supposed to do?" "What did I just say to you?" Ask these questions in a loving, affirmative tone—not one that is condescending and degrading.
- Provide your child with simple puzzles, I-spy books, and toys that produce visible results.

Children with Tourette's and Epilepsy:

- Make sure your child takes their medication on schedule.
- Have regular medical checkups and evaluations.
- Make sure everyone in the family, teachers, and caregivers know what to do in the event of a seizure.
- Educate those who live and work with your child on the facts about Tourette's, Epilepsy, or other neurological disorder.
- Remember that the vast majority of children with Tourette's and Epilepsy have no mental or emotional disabilities. They are what society considers high-functioning children.
- Children with Epilepsy should always wear helmets when riding a bike or skating.

- Never allow an epileptic child to swim alone or be left alone in the tub. Older children should not be allowed to take a bath...showers only.
- Make sure your child has a medical alert bracelet or necklace on in the event they require emergency care and you are not with them. This will allow those around them to get the help your child needs.

REMEMBER: Awareness and knowledge are your child's two best allies when it comes to living with and thriving in spite of their special needs.

Bible Verses to Encourage You

You also, as living stones, are being built up a spiritual house, a holy priesthood, to offer up spiritual sacrifices acceptable to God through Jesus Christ. 1 Peter 2:5 (NKJV)

Be anxious for nothing, but in everything by prayer and supplication, with thanksgiving, let your requests be made known to God; and the peace of God, which surpasses all understanding, will guard your hearts and minds through Christ Jesus. ~Philippians 4:6-7

*Take heed that ye despise not one of these little ones; for I say unto you, that in heaven **their** angels do always behold the face of my Father which is in heaven. ~Matthew 18:10*

Chapter 9: Dealing with Genetic and Physical Special Needs

Among the most common physical and genetic problems facing parents of children with special needs include: cystic fibrosis, multiple sclerosis, cerebral palsy, downs syndrome, congenital birth defects of the vital organs or limbs, dyslexia, and muscular dystrophy.

There are of course, less common and even rare forms of these types of diseases and disorders including, dwarfism and SMA (spinal muscular atrophy)—to name just a few. And then there are those families dealing with special needs resulting from accidental injuries and problems resulting from the birth mother's abuse of drugs and alcohol.

No matter what the cause of the defect, disease, or injury, the fact remains that a child needs and deserves to enjoy the highest quality of life possible.

Therefore, it is the wise and caring parent who makes the most of every opportunity and resource to help make that happen. You can be that parent when you:

- No matter what your child's special needs are, make sure everyone who lives with and spends time with your child on a regular basis knows what your child's condition is, what their needs are, has a working knowledge of how to meet those needs, and knows what to do in an emergency as well as how to do it.
- Make sure your child receives regular checkups and evaluations by their doctor and specialists.
- Make sure your child gets adequate rest, exercise (to the best of their ability), and social and intellectual stimulation and interaction.

- Make sure your child is eating a healthy and nutritious diet. Make this a family thing. For example: If your child is diabetic, don't make them feel deprived and different by keeping candy in the house for everyone else. Make it a special treat for everyone—even your diabetic on occasion.
- Be your child's advocate by taking whatever steps are necessary to ensure they receive the education they deserve and the assistance they need to reach their full potential.
- Do your homework. Stay up on the news concerning available resources for your child.

- Realize there are some things your child simply cannot do. When this happens you need to remember two things: 1) don't make your other children miss out on things. Let them enjoy the life they have been given. And 2) don't make a big deal out of it. Instead, focus on the things they *can* do and let them give those things 100%.

Children with Downs's Syndrome

- Embrace and enjoy their loving, affectionate nature.
- Encourage them to participate in social activities.
- Make sure they are receiving the best possible balance of mainstream classroom learning and classes targeted to meet their special needs. Downs kids are not dumb. They just need help learning how to express and use what they know.

- Parents of children with downs need to make exercise and healthy eating a priority to combat their tendency to be overweight and have heart problems.

Children with mobility needs

- Take your child for regular medical checkups and evaluations. Most mobility diseases and defects are progressive in nature; meaning they only get worse over time. You and your child need to know what is going on inside their body in order to meet their changing needs.
- Establish a regular routine for physical therapy. Movement of the right kind is essential for maintaining a quality of life for your child.
- Make sure your home is fully accessible to them. No child should feel unwelcome or in the way in their own home.

- Make sure your home is a safe place for your child. Loose rugs, exposed cords, and furniture that is unsteady can be hazardous.
- Equip your home in such a way that your child can grow into an independent young person. Make sure they can access the microwave and stovetop. Make sure the refrigerator opens in the direction necessary for them to be able to reach things easily. Make sure light switches are reachable. Lower the rods and shelves in their closet. Install a shower or tub to accommodate their needs with minimal or no assistance.

- Provide forms of exercise and entertainment they can enjoy at home: a swing set to accommodate their needs, a hot tub (ONLY with adult supervision), fuse ball, games with little or no physical movement required (trivia, etc.), audio books, and special instruments that will allow them to work the computer, and telephone.
- Take family outings that are wheelchair-friendly. Most state and national parks and sites are, as well as city parks, theaters, and amusement parks.

Children with genetic and other physical limitations

Genetic abnormalities can show themselves physically, mentally, or emotionally. The degree to which they show themselves also varies widely; ranging from things like dyslexia to an inability to speak or breathe without the assistance of a machine.

Because there are so many different forms or levels of special needs your child might have because of these things, it is important that you educate yourself as much as possible in regards to:

- The particulars of your child's needs and condition
- The resources available to you and your child
- What you can and cannot expect in the way of progression or digression
- What you should and shouldn't expect of your child
- How to properly care for your child
- How to help your child reach their full potential

When it's all is said and done, the most important thing you can remember as the parent of a special-needs child is that Jesus loves the little children - ALL the little children of the world – And that means Your Child too.

Bible Verses to Encourage You

Lo, children are a heritage of the Lord: and the fruit of the womb is His reward.
~Psalm 127:3

Behold the fowls of the air: for they sow not, neither do they reap, nor gather into barns; yet your heavenly Father feedeth them. Are ye not much better than they? ~Matthew 6:26

*for I was hungry and you gave Me food; I was thirsty and you gave Me drink; I was a stranger and you took Me in; I was naked and you clothed Me; I was sick and you visited Me; I was in prison and you came to Me. "Then the righteous will answer Him, saying, 'Lord, when did we see You hungry and feed You, or thirsty and give You drink? When did we see You a stranger and take You in, or naked and clothe You? Or when did we see You sick, or in prison, and come to You?' And the King will answer and say to them, **'Assuredly, I say to you, inasmuch as you did it to one of the least of these My brethren, you did it to Me.'**.*
~Matthew 25:35-40

Chapter 10: Your Not-So-Secret Secret Thoughts

As the parent of a special-needs child you have thoughts and feelings parents of other kids don't have. You think:

- Why my child? Why don't they get to run and play? Why can't they enjoy something as simple as licking an ice cream cone or sloshing through a mud puddle in their bare feet? Why do they have to be the one kids make fun of and shy away from?
- Why doesn't God answer my prayers to heal my child? He healed all those other people in the Bible?
- If I hear the term 'short bus', 'retard', or 'freak' one more time I'm going to explode all over whoever says it.

- I just wish I could have one day that was the kind of normal most people have.
- I know they say it's not my fault, but...but...is it...maybe?

And yes, some of you have even thought:

- If we wouldn't have had this to deal with, our marriage would have survived.
- It's not fair to my other children for me to have to devote so much of myself to their sibling.
- My husband or wife and I are never going to know what it's like to be just the two of us.
- What's going to happen to him/her when we can no longer take care of him/her? Who will take over?
- I'm so tired I don't know if I can do this again tomorrow.

You are only human, so it is natural for you to become weary, worried, and worn down. But the great news is—the news you *have to hold tight to*—is that you don't have to remain weary, worried, and worn down. God the Father, Jesus the Son, and the Holy Spirit are here to help. They are here to take these things from you and replace them with rest, peace, and hope.

As we close out our 'time' together, I want to leave you with some final words of encouragement from the scripture. My prayer is that these words will inspire you to be thankful for and mindful of the fact that you have been chosen by God to care for and rise up one of his extra-special children.

God bless you abundantly!

Bible Verses to Encourage You

Casting down arguments and every high thing that exalts itself against the knowledge of God, bringing every thought into captivity to the obedience of Christ; ~2 Corinthians 10:5

Finally, brethren, whatever things are true, whatever things are noble, whatever things are just, whatever things are pure, whatever things are lovely, whatever things are of good report, if there is any virtue and if there is anything praiseworthy—meditate on these things. ~Philippians 4:8

I beseech you therefore, brethren, by the mercies of God, that you present your bodies a living sacrifice, holy, acceptable to God, which is your reasonable service. And do not be conformed to this world, but be transformed by the renewing of your mind, that you may prove what is that good and acceptable and perfect will of God. ~Romans 12:1-2

Special Gift

God has a Gift for You!   The Plan of Salvation:

There is no formal prayer of salvation as many churches would have you believe, God's Word is very clear - there is only one way to get to the Father in heaven and that is through Jesus Christ (John 14:6). Jesus says that you must be born again to enter into heaven (John 3:3-5).

Salvation is simply the first step in building an open and honest relationship with God. We all have sinned and fallen short, but there is Hope in Jesus Christ - Just cry out to God in sincerity and honesty asking for forgiveness and for Him to Save you, Sanctify you, and fill you with His Holy Spirit - Ask for His will to be done in your life on earth as it is in Heaven and That's it, now just keep it real with God.

A Warning:

The Christian walk is not an easy life on the surface. The Word of God says that we will be hated in all the world for Christ namesake (Matt. 24:9). The Bible says that in the last days are enemy prevail against us physically until Christ returns to save us (Dan 7:21, 22). Furthermore, we must endure hardship as a good soldier of Jesus Christ (2 Tim 2:3) and yet we are never alone in this, God promises us that He will never leave us nor forsake us if we believe in him (Matt.28:20).

In everything we go through we have the peace and joy of God which surpasses all understanding (Philp. 4:6-8) The Bible declares, "For I consider the sufferings of this present time are not worthy to be compared with the glory which shall be revealed in us". (Rom 8:18). However, in all these things we are more than conquerors through Jesus Christ (Rom. 8:37)

Stay in Contact

Stay in Contact with the American Christian Defense Alliance, Inc. through Our Website At: ACDAInc.Org

Join Our Mailing List

We also Greatly Appreciate You Signing Up For Our Mailing List and Providing a Good Rating and review for this Book. Your reviews help other people like yourself find this book and benefit from its contents.

If You or Your Family have been Blessed by this book please let us know by dropping us a line through our website at ACDAInc.Org

Find All Our Books

<u>Some of Our Books:</u>

Parenting: How To Be A Great Parent And Raise Awesome Kids

Prayer: Your No. 1 Prayer Book To Learn To Be A Strong Christian Prayer Warrior That Prays With Powerful Prayers In The War Room To Overcome And Defeat The Enemy

Salvation for Your Unsaved Mom: 10 Things to Tell Your Mom Before She Dies

Wisdom from Your Elders: Learning From Your Parents, Grandparents, and the Older People in Your Church

Kids and Prayer: Pray with Your Kids and Teach Them How to Pray

Embracing Pregnancy, Your Child, and Parenting: A Christian Parenting Guide to Offer Encouragement During the Wonders, Joy, and Hope of Your First Child

Race Relations in America: A Christian Guide to Unite Christians in the Faith

Martial Arts Ministry: How To Start A Martial Arts Ministry

Biblical Bug Out: Don't Bug In - Follow The Calling

Christian Prepping 101: How To Start Prepping

How to Finance Your Full-Time RV Dream

Make Money: A Beginners Guide to Start an Online Business, Work from Home, Make Money, and Develop Financial Freedom

Additional Formats

Thank you for reading this book. Your support and the support of others continue to humble us and enable our Ministry to grow. We hope and pray that this book has blessed you in some way. If you enjoyed this book consider purchasing it as a gift for someone who could benefit from it.

We Greatly Appreciate Your Support as Well as You Sharing this information, including links to our books with Others on Your Social Media Platforms

Thank You Once Again for Your Support; We Know God Will Bless You as You Have Blessed This Ministry

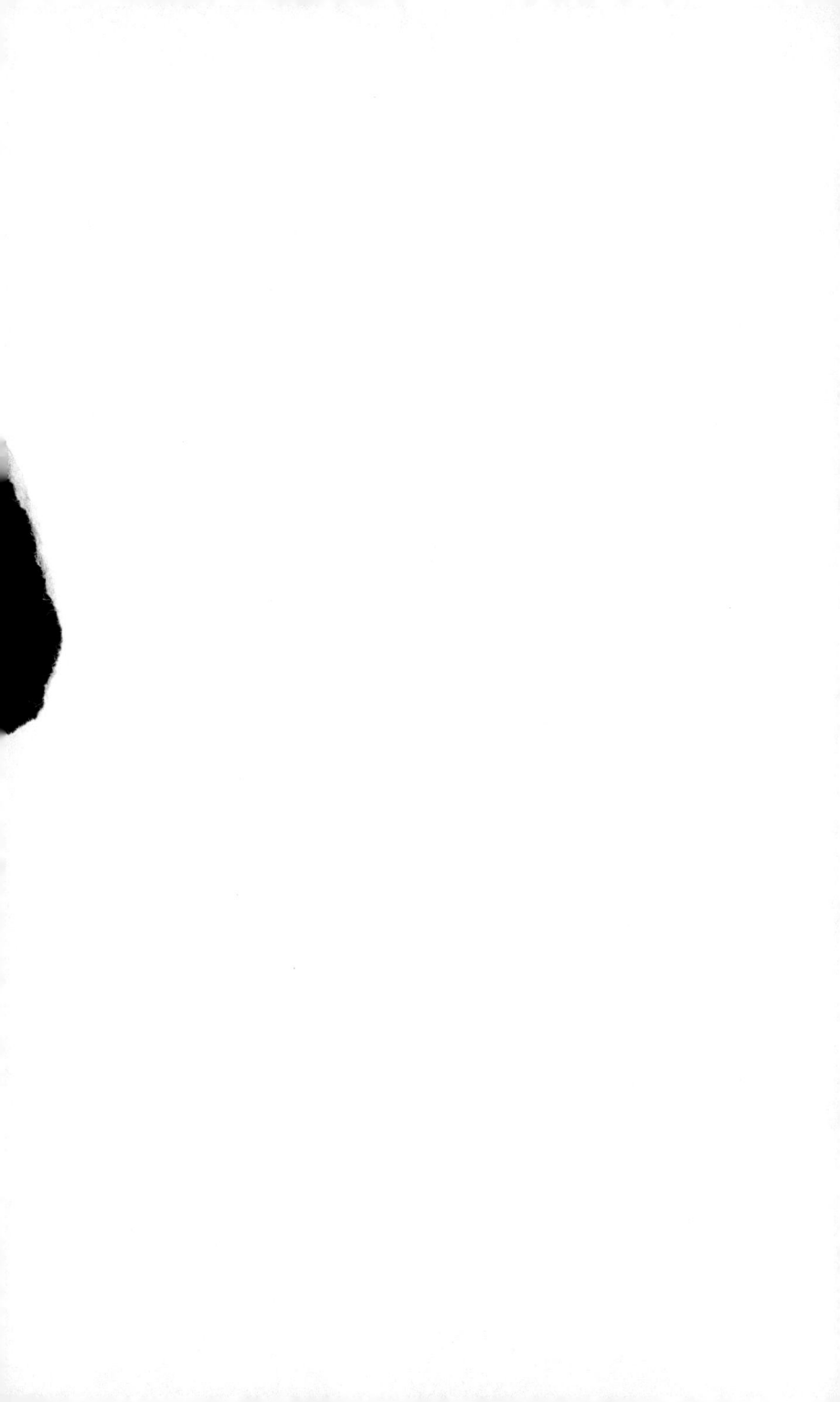

www.ingramcontent.com/pod-product-compliance
Lightning Source LLC
Chambersburg PA
CBHW030939240526
45463CB00015B/408